Cookbook for Candida Diet:

A detailed cookbook for candida

By

Crystal M. Thompson

DISCLAIMER PAGE

Table of Content

INTRODUCTION

Candida's diet foods include non-starchy veggies, low-sugar fruits, lean meats, and fermented foods.

Look for foods that haven't been processed and don't have any added sugars.

Avoid any meals that may cause inflammation, particularly in the stomach. Gluten, alcohol, some vegetable oils, and caffeine are examples of them.

Consume foods that lower inflammation and encourage gut healing, such as fermented foods and bone broth.

The Candida diet is a well-balanced anti-inflammatory diet that may help with gut health, digestion, and immunity. It may also aid in the treatment of Candida symptoms such as yeast infections, tiredness, and food sensitivities.

CHAPTER 1

Changing your eating habits may help you improve your gut health and bring harmony into your life. This action plan and recipes will teach you all you need to know about candida overgrowth and how it impacts your health. You will get a three-step action plan as well as recipes to help you heal your digestive system.

Learn about the physical and mental health difficulties that candida may cause, as well as how your diet can support or prevent its development.

A three-phase wellness plan discovers a realistic approach that will assist you in repairing your gut issues, rebuilding helpful bacteria, and revitalizing yourself.

One of the most difficult aspects of the anti-Candida Diet is determining what to eat. You have a list of items to eat and avoid, but

how do you put all of these new elements together to create a meal?

Here are some ideas for tasty Candida diet recipes:

- Include a variety of fresh veggies.
- Include a couple of low-sugar fruits.
- Stick to non-glutenous grains that are Candida-safe.
- Consume some fermented probiotic foods.
- Caffeine and other stimulants should be avoided.
- Avoid additional sugars, which might feed Candida.
- Use a variety of herbs and spices to season your dishes.
- This section contains a variety of Candida Diet recipes. We're continually adding new items, so keep checking back. There are also some useful tips on utilizing antifungals in your cooking and what to drink instead of coffee in the morning!

Candida Recipe Suggestions

We've compiled a terrific collection of simple (and tasty!) meals that are ALL appropriate with your candida cleanses in this area.

BREAKFAST
Because it's the most important meal of the day, it should be delicious! A nutritious breakfast should include healthy fats, protein, and veggies, like these Avocado Baked Eggs with Vegetable Hash. These nutrients are critical for hormonal signaling and enhancing energy and mood.

Cortisol levels should be at their peak when you get up in the morning. Cortisol is a stress hormone, however, it is important for waking up and staying awake. Eating on a regular schedule is essential for maintaining stable cortisol levels and promoting early-morning energy levels.

LUNCH
Lunch on the Candida diet should be as nutritious and pleasurable as any other meal.

Include the key nutrients: protein and fiber, for example, to help make a balanced meal. This Asian Chicken and Cabbage Salad is very delicious!

Fiber is not just vital for regularity; it also maintains blood sugar levels and decreases cholesterol. That is why naturopaths and certified dietitians advocate consuming at least five grams of fiber every meal. Fiber keeps you full throughout the day, preventing the dreaded ' p.m. slump' that has you reaching for the chocolate cookies!

These delicious meals are high in fiber and protein, which will keep you full and powered all afternoon. And they're so tasty that you'll look forward to lunch break every day!

DINNER
Dinner may be difficult. Overeating - or eating the wrong sorts of food - may disrupt your sleep,

and an unsatisfying meal might lead to reaching for a sugary late-night snack!

A balanced supper includes veggies, protein, fiber, and healthy fat. Nourishing supper ideas like this Curried Chicken Bowl will make you a household favorite!

SNACKS

Snacking between meals is not harmful if done correctly. Healthy snacks like this Mediterranean Zucchini Dip can keep you going until your next meal without disrupting your anti-Candida regimen.

DESSERTS

Who said sweets had to be avoided? Not us!

It's normal to seek a sweet treat from time to time. The key is to fulfill that hunger without succumbing to sweets. Fortunately, many natural sweeteners, such as stevia, xylitol, and monk fruit extract, contain no sugar and have no effect on your blood sugar.

These sweeteners, together with nutritional ingredients like coconut, avocado, and healthy flours, are used in delicious sweets like Coconut Ginger Clouds.

DRINKS

While alcohol is not permitted, healthy beverages are strongly encouraged. Smoothies are a simple and tasty way to eat on the move, and juicing may be a wonderful method to replenish your body with a variety of nutrients all at once. These drink ideas make the most of antimicrobial ingredients while remaining delicious - even this sugar-free eggnog!

Using the Anti-Candida Diet to Restore Gut Health

Poor nutrition is one of the leading causes of Candida overgrowth in the stomach. Sugary meals not only cause inflammation in the body, but they also feed the Candida yeast, enabling it to grow.

Simply follow these Candida diet suggestions to reclaim your gut health, defeat Candida, and return to perfect health!

Consume healthy proteins and fats.
Healthy fats and oils are fantastic methods to maintain gut health, and many of them also have antifungal or anti-inflammatory qualities. Coconut oil, olive oil, butter, and ghee are all excellent choices.
Avoid gluten at all costs.
Avoiding gluten will aid in the healing of your intestines and minimize overall inflammation. It may even help to reverse some of the harm caused by a bacterial imbalance in your stomach. Pseudo-grains like quinoa, buckwheat, and millet are good choices.
Reduce your alcohol consumption.
Alcohol and intestinal permeability are clearly linked. Candida albicans may also induce intestinal permeability, and alcohol exacerbates any gut damage.

Alcohol also destabilizes your blood glucose levels, which may result in unpleasant sugar cravings.

Improve your nutrition.

Low-starch veggies, fruits, and lean meats contain more micronutrients than any other food, making them the greatest choice for a healthy lifestyle. When possible, buy organic and consume a variety of superfoods such as kale, spinach, blueberries, goji berries, fermented foods, and organ meats such as liver.

Drink plenty of water.

Dehydration may cause poor attention, weariness, headaches, low mood, anxiety, and decreased memory, however, drinking water can aid digestion. Drink at least two liters of filtered water every day.

CHAPTER 2

Candida's Diet Eating Habits

What foods should you avoid if you have Candida? If you believe that your stomach is out of balance, the first place to investigate is your food. A high-sugar, processed-food diet may lead to yeast infections, stomach problems, and reduced immunity.

Eating the appropriate meals, on the other hand, helps rebalance your stomach and avoid unpleasant symptoms. By the end of this page, you'll understand precisely how to follow a low-sugar, anti-inflammatory diet that will begin to reset your gut.

We've divided our Candida diet food list into a few simple dietary groupings. The table below contains a list of them. Each food category is described in further depth further down the page.

Many of these foods are very beneficial for supporting gut health and healing from Candida overgrowth.

This website has three Candida food lists. This article contains a list of things to eat. You may also look at the list of foods to avoid (for example, fruit drinks and sugary snacks) and the list of maybe foods (for example, beans, peaches, grains).

- Foods to Consume

It is critical to understand why certain items were selected for the Candida diet. Consider the following three criteria:

Low-sugar

Candida albicans use sugar to grow, infiltrate your gut, and form biofilms that shield it from the immune system . It makes no difference whether the sugars you consume are natural (e.g., bananas) or processed (e.g., candy bars). This list only includes foods with a low sugar content.

- Gluten-free

There is mounting evidence that glutenous meals may cause health concerns in people who are not celiac . Gluten, which is found in bread, pasta, and cereal, may trigger persistent inflammation in your stomach and damage the link between the cells lining your intestinal wall. Our Candida diet food list exclusively includes gluten-free grains and pseudo-grains.

- Anti-inflammatory

One of the most important aspects of the Candida diet is to avoid inflammation. That is why we advise you to avoid processed meals, limit your caffeine intake, and consume plenty of anti-inflammatory, fermented foods.

- Meals That Are Both Healthy and Delicious

Your Candida diet should contain a variety of non-starchy veggies, probiotic foods, lean meats, and non-glutenous grains. You'll be surprised at how many easy, wonderful dinners you can make.

Take a peek at our recipes section for some inspiration!

During your Candida diet, you should be able to consume all of the things on the list in acceptable quantities. If you consume these Candida foods, you can be certain that you are not fueling your Candida overgrowth and that you are making progress toward regaining your health.

This page's foods should make up the bulk of your diet. You may also consume items from the Maybe list, but only in tiny quantities and in a manner that does not enhance their glycemic load.

Keep in mind that your meals should be well-balanced. An egg salad with a basic dressing of olive oil, lemon, and salt is a nice example.

This meal comprises eggs for protein, olive oil for healthy fats, and carbohydrates from avocado and other veggies. Plus a plethora of beneficial vitamins and minerals.

The average American diet is high in carbs, high in processed foods, and poor in nutrients . This is one of the reasons why gut health is so bad in general. If you stick to the Candida diet, you'll be consuming foods that are nutrient-dense, unprocessed, and beneficial to your general health.

CHAPTER 3

List of Candida Diet Foods

Here is a list of items to avoid when on a Candida cleanse:

- Vegetables that are not starchy
- Fruits with low sugar content
- Gluten-free grains
- Proteins that are good for you
- Several dairy products
- Nuts and seeds that are resistant to mold
- Herbs, spices, and sauces
- Oils and fats that are good for you
- Stevia and monk fruit are examples of natural sweeteners.
- Foods that have been fermented
- Chicory coffee and herbal teas are examples of beverages.

Here's a table with a list of Candida foods.

Vegetables that are not starchy
Non-starchy veggies deprive Candida colonies of the natural sugars that sustain them. Consume low-starch veggies such as asparagus, broccoli, eggplant, onions, and zucchini. Fresh veggies should be purchased and consumed raw, steamed, or grilled.

Reduce your intake of starchy vegetables including sweet potatoes, potatoes, yams, maize, winter squash, beets, peas, parsnips, and beans, particularly towards the beginning of your diet. When starting a low-sugar diet, it is common to be tempted to consume a lot of starchy vegetables as a replacement.

Vegetables that are rich in micronutrients but low in carbohydrates are typically the healthiest to consume. All leafy greens, such as spinach or kale, fall under this category.

They also include cruciferous vegetables such as broccoli, cauliflower, and cucumber.

Rutabaga (also known as Swede) is an exemption and is permitted in the diet. Although it is classified as a starchy vegetable, it has a low net carbohydrate content. It is also on our list of antifungal foods, so it may aid in the rebalancing of your gut flora .

Jicama is another notable example. It, like rutabaga, has a low glycemic load and is surprisingly low in net carbs. The nicest thing about jicama is that it is high in inulin, a prebiotic that feeds the 'good bacteria' in your stomach and promotes a healthy gut flora.

It is important to cook your veggies properly. Roasted carrots, for example, have a substantially greater glycemic load than raw or steamed carrots. You may be able to eat raw or cooked carrots without worrying about your blood sugar levels. Fried onions, on the other hand, have a far greater glycemic load than raw onions.

In general, eating your veggies raw or cooked is the best option. Depending on the vegetable, boiling, grilling, gently frying, and roasting are all viable options.

While we're talking about starchy veggies. It's important to remember that you shouldn't be overly rigorous with your diet. You should consume largely from this page's Candida foods list, but you may feel free to include a few things from the Maybe list as well. If you limit your diet too much (e.g., no carbohydrates at all), you may enter a state of ketosis, which might fuel a Candida overgrowth .

Here are some excellent recipes that incorporate the non-starchy veggies on this list.
Patties made with quinoa and rutabaga
Bowl of chicken fajitas
Salad of salmon with arugula dressing

Artichokes cooked in the oven
Salad with buckwheat and Brussels sprouts

When selecting veggies to consume, consider more than simply the carbohydrate content. What you should truly be looking at is something called 'net carbs'. This takes into consideration the fact that not all carbs in your diet will affect your blood sugar in the same way. Fiber and sugar alcohols have minimal influence on blood sugar levels, hence they are avoided.

To determine net carbs, add the entire quantity of carbohydrates to the total amount of fiber and sugar alcohols. As you can see, several high-carbohydrate veggies may have low net carbohydrates if they are rich in fiber.

A good example is Brussels sprouts. A g serving has g of carbs but just g of fiber. That implies a serving has just g of net carbohydrates.

Fruits Low in Sugar

Fruit is normally consumed in limited quantities on the Candida diet. Fruits have a high net carbohydrate content, and some of the natural sugars present in fruits may fuel a Candida overgrowth .

Candida albicans can not distinguish between natural and processed sugars. It can utilize both to sustain its colonies and to form biofilms to defend itself against your immune system.

There are distinctions between the three forms of sugar often present in fruits. Fruits contain varied levels of fructose, glucose, and sucrose, which your body reacts differently.

Sucrose has been demonstrated to significantly promote Candida growth and biofilm formation . It has also been shown that glucose promotes Candida albicans growth and activity .

Fructose is a unique sugar. According to research, Candida metabolizes fructose more slowly than other sugars . Furthermore, there is evidence that fructose may suppress the development of Candida albicans . In fact, fructose is still sometimes prescribed as a diabetic sweetener .

Of course, there is a difficulty. Long-term fructose consumption may result in insulin resistance, fatty liver disease, diabetes, and other health problems.
However, if you maintain a low-sugar diet and avoid fructose-based sweets, this should not be an issue.
What does this all imply for Candida's diet of fruits? When determining which fruits to include in your diet, you need to consider two factors. To begin, remove the fiber and sugar alcohols from the carbohydrates to get the total carbs. Second, determine how much of those sugars are made up of fructose, glucose, and sucrose.

Remember that fructose has a lower influence on blood sugar than the other two natural sugars.

Some fruits, such as lemons, limes, and avocado, have minimal effect on blood sugar levels. You can definitely eat them while on the Candida diet. Others, such as grapes, bananas, and figs, are rich in net carbohydrates and so unsuitable.

When you first start your Candida diet, stick to foods that are low in natural sugars. Other low-sugar fruits, such as berries or apples, may be consumed in moderation.

Here are a few dishes that make use of low-sugar fruits:
Lemon parsley butter atop avocado pancakes
Muffins with strawberries

Pseudo-grains and Non-Glutenous Grains
Grains and pseudo-grains are one area of the Candida diet where there is considerable debate. Non-glutenous grains, according to some

practitioners, may be ingested in any quantities. Others say that the net carbohydrates in these cereals should be avoided at all costs. The reality lies someplace in between.

Regular grains, such as wheat and barley, should be avoided because of their gluten concentration. Although it was once contentious, it is now widely accepted that gluten may cause health issues in those who do not have celiac disease. Gluten, in fact, has been demonstrated to activate the systemic immune system and harm the gut lining .

If you have a persistent Candida overgrowth in your intestine, your gut is most certainly already affected. Allow it to repair itself by avoiding gluten, and consider consuming gut-healing nutrients and foods. L-glutamine, slippery elm, and marshmallow root are all good examples.

The issue of net carbohydrates is more complex. Pseudo-grains like buckwheat, millet, and quinoa don't contain gluten, but they do have a high net carbohydrate content. g of buckwheat groats, for example, has g of net carbohydrates. Normally, this would rule them out of a Candida diet. However, they offer various health advantages that offset the net carbohydrates.

Let's look at buckwheat in more detail. This extraordinary pseudo-grain (really a fruit seed) offers several health advantages. It decreases inflammation, cholesterol, and blood pressure, and may even protect against cancer . It also has prebiotic properties that help support healthy gut flora, which is essential to the Candida diet .

Quinoa, other millets, and amaranth have also been demonstrated to contain prebiotics, which helps feed the healthy bacteria that already exist in the gut .

Overall, the health-promoting and prebiotic properties of these pseudo-grains exceed their rather high net carbohydrate content. They should, however, be used in moderation.

A classic Candida diet error is to concentrate on one thing on the list and consume massive quantities of it. These pseudo-grains may be a modest element of a well-balanced anti-Candida diet, but only in limited amounts.

We should also talk about the flours made from these pseudo-grains. In general, grinding anything into flour will likely slightly enhance its influence on your blood sugar. Treat these flours with prudence and, once again, consume in moderation. If you wish to bake, combine them with other flours with lower net carb counts. Coconut flour and almond flour are two good examples.

Here are a few recipes that use pseudo-grains:
Quinoa from Thailand

Breakfast muffins made with buckwheat
Bowl of satay chicken

Meat, seafood, and eggs
Protein is an essential component of any diet, but it is especially crucial in the Candida diet. When you limit carbs, the calories you lose must come from a mix of fats and protein. Cutting carbs may be a significant shift, but keep in mind that this is not a weight reduction plan. Even if you're eating less carbohydrates, you should still make sure you're getting enough calories.

When purchasing proteins, there are a few things to bear in mind.

Look for meals that are high in nutrients and as fresh as possible.
This might include purchasing organic or local products, or just dealing with a reputable butcher or fisherman.
Avoid adding anything to your meats.

Dextrose, nitrates, and sulfates are common examples. Processed meats should be avoided entirely (don't believe anybody who tells you that bacon is healthy!)

Keep an eye out for pollutants in fish.

Toxin levels in certain fish are much greater than in others. The most often stated examples are tuna and swordfish . Toxins (especially mercury and other heavy metals) may impair your immune system, making you more susceptible to diseases like Candida.

Eggs are your ally.

Organic, free-range eggs are the best source of protein. Eggs are a nutritious powerhouse, and you should feel OK eating several each day if you want.

Limit your consumption of red meat.

If you want to consume red meat, be aware of the negative effects it may have on your digestion and overall health. Red meat may induce constipation and has been related to numerous gastrointestinal malignancies.

Limit your consumption and, wherever feasible, seek pasture-raised, hormone-free meat.

Don't forget about the bone broth.

If you've been suffering from Candida overgrowth, your stomach probably needs some help. Candida has been demonstrated to cause damage to the gut lining, which may lead to other symptoms such as food allergies. Bone broth includes collagen, glutamine, glycine, and proline, all of which may assist in restoring intestinal health (,).

Here are some delectable dishes that include meat, fish, or eggs:

Meatballs made with kimchi

Piccata di chicken

Baked eggs in a skillet

Salad with Nicoise sardines

Milk and dairy products

Fermented dairy products are the finest to consume. Live probiotic cultures aid in the repopulation of your gut with beneficial bacteria, while the fermentation process decreases the sugar level of the meal. There are two excellent examples of probiotic dairy foods that you may include in your Candida diet.

Perhaps the most widely accessible probiotic food is probiotic yogurt. It is widely available in supermarkets, frequently under various brand names. Make sure it includes live cultures when you purchase it; it should state so somewhere on the box. Also, look for yogurt with no added sugar or flavorings. You're searching for plain, probiotic yogurt.

Kefir is a specialty item that is fast growing in popularity. If you've never had it, it's a milk-based fermented drink that tastes like a tangier form of yogurt. Kefir often has a distinct collection of probiotic microorganisms from yogurt. There's no reason you can't include both in your diet.

Here is a list of probiotic strains that are often found in milk kefir. It's worth noting that they

include some types of helpful yeast (not all yeasts, like Candida albicans, are opportunistic pathogens!).
One of the benefits of fermented dairy products is that they may be made at home. Making your own yogurt or kefir is a simple process that everyone can accomplish.

Other dairy products are more difficult to understand. Because butter and ghee are low in lactose (particularly ghee), they are OK. Some cheeses, especially those low in lactose, may be OK on the Candida diet, although they still contain significant levels of casein. Because of the lactose and casein content, milk is often avoided. Lactose is a natural sugar, whereas casein is a protein that causes many dairy allergies.

Also, organic dairy products are a far better option. Non-organic dairy products often include hormones and antibiotics, which may disrupt the stomach and inhibit long-term healing.

Here are a few recipes that include fermented dairy products:
Yogurt parfait with apples and walnuts
florets of buffalo cauliflower
Zucchini dip with a Mediterranean twist

Seeds and nuts
Nuts are a healthful method to increase your calorie intake now that you've committed to eating less carbohydrates.

Most nuts are low in carbohydrates, and serving sizes are typically tiny. There are a few nuts that are rich in net carbohydrates (cashews and pistachios, for example), so be cautious while eating them. Pecans and Brazil nuts have the lowest net carbohydrate content.

Mold is another factor to consider while discussing nuts. Most nuts contain at least some mold, which may be problematic for Candida patients. This is not due to mold 'feeding the

Candida,' as you may have heard elsewhere. Candida patients are very susceptible to mold exposure, and the mold in the nuts may cause a response.

. Many Candida dieters consume a lot of nuts and have no problems. They are an essential element of the diet for vegetarians in particular.

If you are worried about mold contamination from the nuts you are eating, soak them in water overnight. Alternatively, spray them with Grapefruit Seed Extract, an antifungal that will swiftly eliminate any remaining mold. Mold is most often seen in cashews, peanuts, and pistachios.

Almond flour and coconut flour are both healthy baking choices with extremely minimal net carbohydrates. They are often blended with a pseudo-grain flour, such as buckwheat.

Here are some recipes that use nuts and seeds:
Smoothie with almonds and mint
Tart crust made with almonds and coconut
Crumb cakes with cinnamon and pecans
Muesli with bircher berries

Condiments, Herbs, and Spices
There are many reasons why herbs and spices should be included in your Candida diet.

For starters, they enhance the taste of your cuisine. This is particularly critical if you've been consuming a lot of processed food till now. When you eliminate hazardous flavorings from your diet, such as high fructose corn syrup and MSG, herbs and spices may replace the void. It might be as simple as sprinkling basil pesto on your chicken.

Second, herbs and spices provide a plethora of additional health advantages.

They may decrease inflammation, promote circulation, assist your liver, and much more, in addition to having almost no carbs.

Good-grade herbs and spices are not always available at your local grocery. The spices there have most likely been bottled and preserved for an extended period of time, frequently more than a year. The spices are stale, maybe moldy, and have lost most of their taste and health advantages at that time.

Ethnic stores and spice merchants are good locations to buy herbs and spices. They are also available from trustworthy sources online. Look for a place with a large turnover; its herbs and spices will most likely be fresher and of greater quality.

Let's look at a few of the spices that you may add to your Candida foods-to-eat list and how they can help battle Candida overgrowth.

Turmeric is a culinary spice with extraordinary health-promoting effects. Curcumin, its major constituent, has been demonstrated to be a powerful antioxidant, decrease inflammation, and aid in the treatment of illnesses such as metabolic syndrome . It is also an antifungal that has been demonstrated to impede Candida albicans growth .

Here are some turmeric-infused recipes:

Grilled chicken in coconut milk with bok choy

Patties made with quinoa and rutabaga

Another notable example is cinnamon. It possesses antifungal activities that have been shown in the lab and in vivo . It may also assist diabetics with blood sugar levels to enhance their glycemic control .

Here are some cinnamon-infused recipes:

Crumb cakes with cinnamon and pecans

Crispy cinnamon coconut

Condiments are more difficult to understand. The vast majority, if not all, of the condiments at your store are very harmful. Condiments like ketchup and HP sauce are high in added sugars, which may fuel a Candida overgrowth, not to mention all the preservatives and colorings that can negatively impact your health.

On the Candida diet, there are no clear alternatives for ketchup. You probably won't miss it if you season your dish properly and use a lot of herbs and spices. Try some coconut aminos if your cuisine needs a little additional flavor. This is similar to soy sauce, however, it is made completely of coconut.

Combine apple cider vinegar, olive oil, lemon, and coconut aminos to make salad dressings. Whatever salad you're making, you may prepare a delectable dressing to bring out the taste of those fresh, delightful ingredients.

Oils and Fats

Not all oils are made equal when it comes to the Candida diet. Canola oil and vegetable oil, for example, are extensively processed and lack many of the nutrients that you would expect from an oil. Other oils, particularly sunflower oil, are heavy in omega- fatty acids, which may be pro-inflammatory unless balanced by a high intake of omega-s.

On a Candida diet, there are many healthful oils that are ideal alternatives. They appear often in the recipes on this page. The finest examples are coconut oil and olive oil, both of which are excellent choices due to their antifungal characteristics.

Olive oil is the most adaptable and beneficial oil to use in your new diet. It includes oleuropein, a powerful component that may inhibit Candida from sticking to the gut membrane . Other studies have shown that it may also lower blood sugar levels . You can use olive oil for baking, cooking, salad dressing, and just about everything else.

When purchasing olive oil, opt for one branded 'extra virgin.' Be careful that there is widespread fraud in the olive oil business, and many bottles may include inferior oils like canola . Find a bottle from a trustworthy brand (Italian producers are the worst, sadly). Even better, seek a local olive oil specialty shop, which is popping up in most major towns and cities.

Coconut oil contains three medium-chain fatty acids: caprylic acid, capric acid, and lauric acid. These wonderful fatty acids have been demonstrated to act together to be effective against Candida albicans when ingested as a whole-food supplement . Coconut oil may be used as a conventional cooking oil or in baking. Keep in mind that it is often solid at room temperature, thus it cannot be used for salad dressings.

In the dairy area, we've previously covered butter and ghee. They are absolutely appropriate for Candida's diet cooking and baking choices.

Sweeteners

When combating a fungal Candida infection, the most crucial thing to eliminate from your diet is added sugar. Candida albicans use sugar to proliferate, spread its colonies, and form a biofilm to shield itself from your immune system.

You should avoid adding sugar to your baking, recipes, or beverages while on the Candida diet. You should also avoid any items with added sweets, such as candy bars, sushi rolls, and processed cereal.

It's difficult to give up sweet foods, particularly if you've had a sweet tooth your whole life! Long term, the idea is to begin loving salty meals and tastes; ultimately, you'll discover that many of your previous favorites are just too sweet for your palette.

For the time being, though, here are three Candida-friendly sweeteners.

Stevia is a zero-calorie natural sweetener with a very sweet taste . In reality, a minimal quantity of stevia is required to replace a spoonful of sugar. The flavor has a little bitterness to it, which some people dislike, yet many Candida dieters use stevia in their cuisine on a daily basis.

For millennia, monk fruit extract has been used as both a sweetener and a medicinal. It's really sweet, just like stevia. However, it lacks stevia's aftertaste and does not induce digestive discomfort like certain sugar alcohols. Monk fruit extract provides no carbohydrates or calories and nothing that might support a Candida infestation.

Following that are erythritol and xylitol. Both of these are sugar alcohols that may be used to sweeten meals without adding carbs to your diet.

Both are suitable for a Candida diet and have been used to control blood sugar levels. Xylitol has also been demonstrated to inhibit Candida albicans acetaldehyde synthesis .

Stevia, erythritol, and xylitol may be used in lieu of sugar, although their effects on blood sugar levels are substantially lower. Because they taste considerably sweeter than sugar, you only need a small amount of these sweeteners. These sweeteners are very beneficial in baking.

Foods that have been fermented
We've previously discussed a number of dairy-based fermented foods, yogurt, and kefir, but fermented foods deserve their own category. Restoring a healthy balance of bacteria in the gut is a critical component of any Candida treatment approach. Probiotic foods may assist you in doing this.

Let's look at some of the greatest fermented foods to include in your Candida diet.

Yogurt is the most popular fermented food, but you must be cautious which yogurt you select. Check to see whether your yogurt has live probiotic strains; it should indicate 'live cultures' and 'probiotic' anywhere on the label. Also, look for yogurt with no added sugar or flavorings. Plain, probiotic yogurt with no added flavors is the best yogurt for Candida.

Kefir is a fermented food that is becoming more popular. It's a fermented milk drink that tastes comparable to (but a touch more sour than) yogurt. Kefir often contains more probiotic strains than yogurt, but both are excellent alternatives for fermented dairy products. They are simple to make at home and need very little equipment.

Let's move on to the fermented dishes made from vegetables. You've undoubtedly had sauerkraut, a basic fermented food made just with cabbage and salt. Sauerkraut is high in probiotic strains and a simple meal to include in your diet. Simply add a scoop to your dish for lunch and supper.

Just be cautious while purchasing sauerkraut from a store. The majority of commercial sauerkrauts are pickled rather than fermented. That is, rather than the time-consuming fermentation procedure, many manufacturers just add vinegar to the cabbage. This sauerkraut has no probiotic microorganisms at all. Examine the labels once again. Words like fermented, living cultures, and probiotics should be included.

Another notable example is olives. When properly fermented, they are a low-carbohydrate fruit accompanied by a plethora of probiotic bacteria that may aid in gut rebalancing. However, unlike sauerkraut, most olives sold in supermarkets are just pickled in vinegar and not fermented.

Drinks
There are however other solutions if you truly miss caffeine or want to gradually wean yourself off of coffee. Green tea is minimally caffeinated

and includes L-theanine, which counteracts the effects of coffee and relaxes you. Matcha is a powdered variant of green tea that has the same effect as green tea but contains additional antioxidants.

If you consume tea, go for organic brands if feasible. Tea and coffee are two of the most pesticide-laden consumables consumed in North America, compromising gut health.

Other beverages on the maybe list include decaffeinated coffee, nut milk, and vegetable juices. Check the net carbohydrates in any juice or milk you purchase, since there are significant changes across brands and kinds.

Here are some beverages that you may create while on the Candida diet:
Smoothie made with coconut
Smoothie with almonds and mint
Tea with turmeric

CHAPTER 4

Candida Could Be Ruining Your Social Life in Ways

As you are surely aware, intestinal Candida overgrowth is unpleasant. Candida may have a number of unpleasant impacts on your social life, in addition to the apparent stomach discomforts and their influence on your health.

The longer you allow a yeast overgrowth to develop in your gut and elsewhere, the worse these symptoms might get – and the more conscious you will be of them in social circumstances.

Here's a rundown of the issues you can be having as a consequence of Candida overgrowth.

Candida Symptoms That Affect Your Social Life

- **BAD BREATHING**

Bad breath makes social interactions very unpleasant. It's tough to talk to someone whose breath makes you want to vomit!

Bad breath, often known as halitosis, is a disorder caused by bacteria in the mouth and stomach. Bad breath may also be caused by opportunistic yeast, such as Candida albicans, according to research.
Although we all have odor-causing bacteria in our lips, those who have persistent bad breath often have a microbiota imbalance in their stomach. This is what causes the microorganisms that cause foul breath to proliferate.

The first step in curing foul breath is to address the bacterial and yeast imbalance in the stomach. Probiotics and a high-fiber diet will assist.

- **PROBLEMS WITH DIGESTION**

Running to the restroom every few minutes is a guaranteed way to ruin a nice night out. Having gas troubles is equally as unpleasant - and incredibly unprofessional for your organization!

Candida overgrowth is a frequent cause of digestive problems such as flatulence, diarrhea, and cramps. When your stomach is bloated, it's also difficult to enjoy a meal or a discussion.

Candida causes gas and bloating by disrupting the balance of your intestinal flora, resulting in excessive fermentation in the gut. A sugary diet can aggravate this, causing painful swelling and bloating.

- ENVIRONMENTAL ALLERGIES/SENSITIVITIES

Do you often sneeze, itch, or break out in a rash for no apparent reason? A yeast imbalance in your stomach might be creating sensitivity to ordinary scents and substances such as perfumes, animal dander, pollen, or specific meals.

There is compelling evidence that gut abnormalities (often referred to as dysbiosis) are associated with undesired immunological responses such as seasonal allergies. In fact, persons who suffer from seasonal allergies are more likely to have less diversified gut microbiota dominated by a few species.

- SLUGGISHNESS AND FATIGUE

A common symptom of Candida overgrowth is feeling weary, sluggish, and 'foggy' all of the time. You may be healthy and have enough of sleep, but a gut imbalance like Candida can sap your vitality to the point that you don't want to do anything sociable!

Candida fatigue is caused by an imbalance of bacteria in the gut. A yeast overgrowth hinders your body's 'good' bacteria from absorbing and breaking down essential elements including vitamins, minerals, and amino acids. Digestion also slows, which may result in extra fermentation in the stomach and further pain.

- IMPROPER MEMORY

Poor memory, like weariness, is very detrimental to your social life. Constantly losing knowledge may cause a variety of embarrassments. Inflammation in the body is often the cause of poor memory. Candida often begins in the gastrointestinal tract. This inflammation affects neurons in the brain and elsewhere to work less effectively, slowing mental sharpness, information retention, and reflexes.

Slow neurons may also limit energy generation in brain cells, causing weariness. This might make it difficult to concentrate on anything.

- ANXIETY AND DEPRESSION

Feeling down or sad is a significant barrier to socializing. Unfortunately, it is also a common Candida symptom.

This is related to the gut-brain connection, which states that many of the disruptions generated by bacterial imbalance in the stomach have a direct impact on mood and cognition.

Many of the hormones involved in mood regulation are known to be produced in the intestine. This contains to % of serotonin, one of the most essential neurotransmitters involved in mood regulation. When yeast overgrowth occurs in the stomach, it may decrease serotonin and other neurotransmitter synthesis. As a consequence, you may have feelings of depression, anxiety, and overall malaise.

- SEX LIFE DISRUPTION

Candida, in addition to hurting your mood, may severely impair your sexual desire. Yeast infections are one source of this, but they may also induce undesired hormonal changes.

Candida overgrowth in the stomach interferes with the synthesis of several hormones, including sex hormones. This may result in lower estrogen and testosterone levels. Because these hormones are closely tied to libido, it's not unusual to have decreased sex desire as a consequence.

Low insulin production may also have an impact on sex hormone and growth hormone production. Growth hormone (GH) is required for normal libido.

Take charge of Candida before it takes control of you.
The many unpleasant symptoms of yeast overgrowth might seriously impair your willingness to socialize with others. When you're weary, gassy, or sad, it's generally better to remain at home.

Take control of your life by addressing the source of your symptoms: Candida overgrowth.

Several vitamins might aid you in your fight against Candida. They work together to remove Candida toxin, restore gut flora, and suppress Candida albicans development.

www.ingramcontent.com/pod-product-compliance
Lightning Source LLC
Chambersburg PA
CBHW071108260726
48661CB00006B/2533